Conquer Your Tinnitus

Understanding and Healing Tinnitus the Natural Way

Table of Contents

Introduction

Panic-stricken, I tightly clenched my entire body and clawed desperately at the sides of my head, begging that incessant banging and whistling to quieten down and leave me alone.

Why won't it stop? What's happening inside there, inside my head? I have a brainaneurysm, I'm sure of it...Maybe I'm going mad... I really could be going crazy here, and there's nobody here to help...pleeeease stop!

I believed I was either losing my mind, or suffering from a huge, life-threatening medical catastrophe, and that this was the end.

But sadly this wasn't too far from the truth. This event was to be huge and life-threatening and catastrophic, but I wasn't dying nor going mad. I had developed tinnitus.

And I really couldn't cope; there was no escape from its clutches.

From that fateful moment that I awoke from a headache-induced nap, right to the moment I was 'cured', it never stopped, not for a single second. It demanded my attention when I tried to concentrate during critical work meetings, irritated when I relaxed with my favorite paperback in the evening, it screamed when I slid into the bath and it hammered right on when I tried to drop off to sleep at night. It was utterly slow torture and it had appeared right out of the blue.

I was convinced it was going to ruin my life. It had already made my life unbearable and I simply wanted to escape.

I went to the emergency room, my doctor and even a specialist and they all gave me the same old well-worn prognosis. *"There is no treatment,"* they each said, *"Go home and be patient. Your symptoms will probably subside in time..."*

So what's a girl to do? Be brave and cling on desperately whilst the days, weeks, months or even years tick by in the hope that 'someday' I might be cured? Try to cope whilst watching life pass me by?

That simply wasn't my style. With a whole lot of grit and determination, I set to helping myself. I researched hour after hour, I spoke to anyone who had facts or suggestions to offer me on my quest and I tried countless treatments from over-the-counter medication to elimination diets, right to acupuncture.

Yet nothing worked for long, and it felt like I was doomed to carry out this life-sentence.

That is, until I stumbled across the answer, and it's surprisingly simple. I am going to share it with you right here, right now so you can feel the same benefits as I have.

By using a combination of approaches from great food to stress relief and therapies, we will attack your tinnitus symptoms from all sides and help you to get some relief from your living hell. How does that sound?

This book is organized in two sections. The first section will tell you all you need to know about tinnitus, what causes it and what is happening within your body during an episode of tinnitus. Then the second section will explain to you the wonderful treatments and techniques that I have personally used to find my 'cure'. It's true that I do still have the occasional relapse today, but I soon rewind and take myself back through 'the healing process' to get to that renewed state of equilibrium.

There is no 100% guarantee that your symptoms will go completely, but together we will give you a fighting chance to be back to normal and living your life again as quickly as possible. Are you with me?

Let's get started.

SECTION 1: ALL ABOUT TINNITUS

This is the part of the book where we explore everything there is to know about tinnitus. We will explain what tinnitus actually is, what effects it can have on your life and what causes it in the first place. Knowledge is power, as they say.

Chapter 1: What is Tinnitus?

Most of us have experienced a degree of ringing in the ears after an exposure to a loud noise, such as listening to music on full volume, enjoying a rock concert or after spending the night at a loud nightclub. I know I have. Luckily, it soon disappears after a day or two and doesn't impact my life.

However, for many people all over the world, this kind of 'ringing' continues day and night for weeks, months or even years at a time and impacts severely upon that person's life and psychological state, sometimes even resulting in depression and suicide. This is known as tinnitus and it is a horrendous beast to do battle with.

For a tinnitus sufferer, their entire life is haunted incessantly by sounds that aren't really there and never ever go away, whether they're awake or asleep, in the library, at work, walking down the street, enjoying your favorite music. There simply isn't any escape and it feels like you're slowly but surely going mad.

These sounds experienced are often described as ringing, humming, buzzing, hissing, grinding or whistling and can range in pitch from high to low, may be mild and barely noticeable, or even more severe and life-limiting. The sound may even change as time goes by, or come and go as it pleases.

But it's not all bad news; tinnitus isn't necessarily a sign of a serious underlying condition and is relatively common in the general population. In fact, it is said that up to 1 in 10 people suffer from mild tinnitus and 1 in 100 cope with a more severe version. It can be encouraging to know that you're far from being alone in your journey with this beast. This certainly was a fact that helped me. And also, tinnitus often resolves itself eventually, over time.

Chapter 2: The Effects of Tinnitus

When my doctor diagnosed my tinnitus, I felt as if my world had collapsed at my feet.

"There is no cure and that you simply have to learn to live with it as best you can," volunteered my doctor with a shrug of his shoulders.

And so I was given my sentence. There seemed no hope, there seemed no escape and I simply felt as if I was going mad, or on the verge of having a nervous breakdown. Life simply didn't seem worth living. Every last aspect of my life was affected by this menace and I couldn't break free.

The majority of people who suffer with tinnitus end up feeling the same as I used to.

Sleep becomes a huge issue for sufferers and instead of being a wonderful relaxing end to the day, becomes a time to be dreaded. Just when the house is quiet and the whole world is drifting off to sleep, tinnitus attacks and sleep becomes impossible. For many, tinnitus only ever rears its ugly head and becomes noticeable when in complete silence. You're unable to drift off, and once you are asleep you are constantly woken. As a result the quality of your sleep is affected which of course affects your physical and mental health and your entire quality of life. You suffer headaches, nausea and depression and live every moment of your life under a thick fog of exhaustion.

And of course, when you suffer from tinnitus you're constantly distracted and no longer able to concentrate on anything at all with that buzzing invading and dominating your brain. As a result, your focus on even the most mundane of tasks drops to zero and your usually-outstanding performance in both work and leisure slides downwards off the scale.

Attempting to cope with this horrendous challenge makes your stress levels shoot skywards and your psychological well-being take a beating. Aside from the irritation you feel and hostility to the sounds themselves, you simply can no longer function. You're anxious, you're unable to relax and you cannot cope any longer. You might even slip into a dark, hopeless depression or even consider suicide.

But my doctor's lack of apparent concern or understanding of my prognosis wasn't his fault.

After all, he doesn't have first-hand knowledge of the hell that is tinnitus, and to an outsider, tinnitus is just a ringing in the ears and seems like no big deal. But if you are a sufferer like me, you know the truth. You know just how much it affects every part of your life.

Chapter 3: The Mechanics of Hearing

What is your favorite sound in the entire world? For me it's listening to my sister's young son laughing in that beautiful carefree way which is so characteristic of childhood. Let's use this as an example to help explain and understand the biology of tinnitus, and what is going on inside your body when you experience tinnitus symptoms. This will help on many levels; it will help us come to terms with our prognosis, accept the symptoms, reduce its psychological impact and in the long-term, help to improve or even heal symptoms altogether.

You're probably feeling right now that your hearing is 'broken' or you are going mad, and that is a perfectly normal way to be feeling right now. Most people who have experienced tinnitus or even another similar condition feel exactly the same as you.

But this is certainly not the case, and we are obviously hearing *something*, whether it is real or not, so let's take a look into the mechanics of it all so we can shed some light on what is happening inside our bodies and give us back the power to heal.

So let's go back to the example I gave earlier to explain how hearing works. When my sister's son laughs, he creates sound waves which travel through the air towards my ears. My outer ear, the bit that you can see, captures the sound and allows it to travel into the inner ear. These sound waves then hit the eardrum and cause it to vibrate in a way similar to that of a regular musical drum, and then in turn move the three tiny bones of the inner ear.

These sound waves then continue on their journey and enter the cochlea (the part that looks like a snail shell) which is both filled with a liquid and also lined with tiny hairs, which causes the liquid and hairs inside to vibrate. This creates the nerve signals that travel to your brain. And last of all your brain then makes sense of the sound waves that I'm hearing, and I interpret it as his laughter (and smile!).

What happens for the tinnitus sufferer?

Tinnitus is a processing problem in the brain. The irritating sounds that taunt you on a daily basis aren't a sign of impending madness, but are instead a signal that things aren't operating quite as they should be in your brain and your nervous system.

Along with the spinal cord, the brain forms part of your central nervous system. We use our central nervous system to make sense of the world around us through our senses: seeing, hearing, touching, smelling and tasting. The job of our brain is to send and receive messages to and from the outside world to your body through your nerve fibres. And then, of course, we can act accordingly.

But the brain of a tinnitus sufferer is a brain in crisis.

Instead of nerve cells firing as the result of an outside stimulus such as the loud music at a rock concert, they continue to fire long afterwards and simply cannot return to a state of rest. This prolonged state of high alert and irregular firing of nerve cells is what causes you to experience the symptoms of tinnitus.

It happens as a result of either physical damage to your hearing apparatus, or as a result of prolonged neurological stress. Follow me to the next chapter when we will investigate what this means, and explore what might be causing *your* tinnitus.

Chapter 4: What is Causing *Your* Tinnitus?

As you saw in the previous chapter, tinnitus is a symptom of nerve cells misfiring and in a state of constant agitation.

This is all great to know, but it doesn't help us on our quest for understanding, does it? What we really want to understand is what caused this tinnitus to occur in the first place.

Of course, everyone is unique and the causes and triggers can be vast, so for that reason I have compiled the list below of the most common causes of tinnitus. It should help you identify the cause of your own symptoms and increase your understanding. What do you think triggered yours?

Hearing damage or hearing loss (temporary or permanent)

Hearing damage or hearing loss is a common cause of tinnitus. If the cochlea is damaged, or the nerve cells are less responsive or a person experiences an overall hearing loss, their brain will try to compensate for the lack of sounds at a certain frequency, and the person experiences tinnitus.

Many people who either work or have worked in noisy professions such as the construction industry or in factories find their hearing suffers as a result, and tinnitus is one of the likely symptoms.

For younger people, excessive noise is usually the trigger for temporary hearing loss and tinnitus, but thankfully this soon resolves itself. This is the case when we have attended a really loud live music concert, or danced the night away at a really loud nightclub and have some mild degree of tinnitus when we return home which is usually gone by the morning.

However, over time, prolonged excessive noise exposure could damage hearing or cause hearing loss on a permanent basis, so it's important to be careful and protect yourself whenever you can.

Problems with inner ear

At times, tinnitus is a symptom of a more temporary problem that soon resolves itself. Problems such as a build-up of earwax, a middle-ear infection or a perforated eardrum are all common causes. When the infection has been fought off, the eardrum has healed, or the excess wax is removed, things soon return to normal and the tinnitus disappears.

Blow to the head/ head injury

Tinnitus can appear following a blow to the head, otherwise known as a head injury. If you have sustained a head injury, it's important that you get yourself checked out as soon as possible to rule out any more concerning causes for the tinnitus. Even if the blow was relatively weak and without other symptoms, be safe rather than sorry and see your doctor.

Illnesses

Tinnitus can appear as a symptom of another illness such as anemia, hyperthyroidism or Meniere's disease. See your doctor if you suffer from one of these illnesses and you experience symptoms of tinnitus.

Lifestyle

Negative lifestyle choices can also result in tinnitus. The primary offenders are alcohol abuse, substance abuse and solvent abuse, all of which can cause long-lasting damage to your body or even death. If you are dealing with issues surrounding alcohol, substance and solvent abuse, please seek help. There are many people out there who will help you through this difficult time.

Allergies

My own symptoms of tinnitus arose as the result of taking a double dose of aspirin, and it reassured me to hear that this is quite common. Other offenders include antibiotics, diuretics and quinine. Visit your doctor if you think your medication is triggering your tinnitus- you may be able to switch to a different brand of medicine that helps your existing health problems without triggering tinnitus.

Certain food allergies can also trigger episodes of tinnitus, such as caffeine, sugar, wheat, dairy and food additives such as MSG. We'll discuss this in more detail in the forthcoming chapter on healing.

Long term chronic stress

Chronic stress is one of the leading causes of illness in the modern world, and it certainly has a role to play in tinnitus. Stress sends the body into an elevated and prolonged state of fight-or-flight and so the body's nervous system remains at that heightened state of alert, which then triggers random firing of neurons and symptoms of tinnitus. In fact, my closest friend developed tinnitus after a negative and challenging life event, followed by a period of chronic stress. She found that the more stress she was under, the stronger her symptoms were.

Posture

Our posture effects everything about our bodies. Choose good posture and your skeleton and spine is aligned correctly and our organs and tissues can function as nature intended. Choose bad posture and everything is compressed and suffocated.

If the parts being compressed are the blood vessels, nerves and muscles involved with hearing then problems and symptoms of tinnitus can be triggered. This is the simplest of all cases of tinnitus to fix- change position and posture and all symptoms should disappear.

SECTION 2: HEALING YOUR TINNITUS

This book has so far enabled you to understand your tinnitus, what 'type' of tinnitus you are suffering from and importantly, what may have caused it.

In this next section, we will give you a 5 step plan that will enable you to eliminate triggers, improve your overall heath and psychological well-being and eliminate stress in your life naturally, without turning to harsh drugs or treatments.

Plus we will suggest several highly effective techniques and tools that will work with you as an individual to reduce or completely eliminate your symptoms. You will become empowered to tackle these horrendous symptoms and begin to live your life again to its fullest. Sounds great, doesn't it?

The five sections that make up the plan are:

STEP 1.   Diagnose your tinnitus
STEP 2.   Heal the physical causes
STEP 3.   Optimum nutrition
STEP 4.   Stress Reduction and management
STEP 5.   Sound therapy

Follow me now through this section to conquer your tinnitus and reclaim your life.

STEP 1: Diagnose Your Tinnitus

A certain amount of tinnitus is completely normal and most people have experienced it at some time or another, but if your own symptoms haven't cleared up after a few days, you really need to find out what is going on and investigate the root cause. Before you do anything else, make sure you visit your GP for a through check.

Your doctor will check your ears, neck and head to investigate the cause of your tinnitus and rule out any underlying medical problems. This will likely involve a through discussion of your symptoms and a hearing examination test to make sure you can explain to your doctor exactly when you started to experience symptoms, what 'types' of sounds they are (ie. humming, buzzing, musical, etc.) and when they change or become more noticeable. If the doctor wants to investigate further, he or she may refer you to a specialist or order some imaging tests such as a MRI or CT scan.

Once your tinnitus has been diagnosed, your doctor should also be able to explain the condition to you in more detail as well as suggesting additional help, treatments or therapy.

STEP 2: Heal the Physical Cause

Next we need to take the essential steps towards healing these physical triggers of your tinnitus, before we then turn our focus towards healing the rest of your body.

Even if the cause of your tinnitus is unknown there's no need to worry. It's likely that there is nothing too sinister lurking inside your body. Once you have been officially diagnosed, you can take steps towards healing.

You might need to have a course of antibiotics or other medication, you might need an ear irrigation treatment, you might need to correct your hearing loss though surgery of physical means. Whatever it is, do this first.

Perhaps your doctor has informed you that there is nothing that can be done, and tell you that this torturous symptom will resolve itself in time, and that you should just wait.

But he or she is wrong. You can take action to help yourself to heal. You can take control and begin to live your life again. Follow the steps outlined in this plan and you **will** beat that tinnitus.

Tackling the root cause of your tinnitus might be all that it takes to resolve it, and if that is the case, fantastic! For the majority of us, tinnitus will be more stubborn and a whole lot harder to shift, but we can do it.

Next we are going to turn to the power of optimal nutrition and how eating better can resolve that tinnitus.

STEP 3: Optimum Nutrition

Food is vital to human health, so why do we often neglect to pay close enough attention to what we are putting into our bodies? We stuff ourselves with white carbs, processed foods, additives and preservatives, high levels of sugar, fat and thousands of suspect chemicals without a moment's thought as to what it is doing to our bodies.

But this needs to stop right here right now.

We can't continue to gorge ourselves on food-like substances, and we cannot (and should not) continue to neglect our bodies, and our health. And if you don't see why, and are solidly stuck in your own eating habits, here's the deal clincher:

Optimum nutrition can help to resolve your tinnitus and prevent it from reoccurring in the future. What else do you need to know?

Instead of filling up on garbage, we need to make healthy food choices and nourish our bodies with the best, high-quality food that is out there.

Great nutrition supports your body and your mind. It boosts your immune system, helps your body heal illness or injuries and promotes excellent mental health.

Most importantly for us, it will help you to cope with the symptoms of tinnitus, promote a more positive and peaceful mindset and help your body to heal and your nervous system to return to a more normal restful state.

In the following section we will explain how you can eat in an abundant and health-promoting way that will boost your overall health as well as tackling your tinnitus. We will also investigate some of the food and lifestyle choices that can trigger your tinnitus symptoms, and finally we will explain the supplements that can help.

(As a reminder, please understand that we are not licensed physicians, please check our recommendations with your doctor first)

What to eat to boost your health

As a nation we have become so accustomed to food that has been pre-prepared in some way that it's easy to forget what food actually is. It's not the box of mac'n'cheese on your supermarket shelf, it's not that family-sized box of sweetened cereal sitting in your cupboard and it's most certainly not that jar of egg whites lying in your fridge door. All of these so-called foods are so far away from the genuine article, that our ancestors would have a hard time even recognizing them as food.

So let's get back to basics.

It really is that simple. I want you to eat a whole food diet rich in all of the wonderful colors of nature and jam-packed full of nutrients that will support your body and your health. Most importantly, these foods should all be bought from the store in their natural state- no chopping, nor processing, nor extra added *anything*.

Cook 'from scratch' as often as you can, and enjoy the flavors of real food. If you're not feeling to confident and think you might succumb to the temptations of packaged food again, check some cookery books out of the local library or enroll in a cookery course to boost your skills: your health will repay you in the long-term, I promise.

One of the most effective steps I took in my journey towards tackling my tinnitus was adopting a nutrient dense diet such as this. And I found my results were better still when I adopted a high-percentage raw diet. Not everyone will find that this way of eating suits them, and I understand completely, but I do advise that everyone aims to increase their consumption of raw fruit and veg throughout the day- eat more salads and get plenty of fresh fruit, and the rest will take care of itself.

What foods to avoid

There are some foods that can trigger attacks of tinnitus, as well as effecting your overall health and well-being. It's important that we avoid these foods as much as possible to give our bodies a chance to return to a positive state of health, and allow our nervous system to return to a state of rest at last, healing our tinnitus as a result.

These are:

-Salt

Reduce your intake of salt. It restricts your blood vessels and increases blood pressure which can cause your symptoms to worsen.

-Caffeine

Reduce your daily consumption of caffeinated products such as tea, coffee, hot chocolate and energy drinks. These may worsen symptoms of tinnitus by increasing blood pressure and stimulating nerve cell activity. Instead try decaffeinated versions or fruit and herbal teas instead.

-Salicylates

This is the natural pesticide that occurs in many foods. Unfortunately they are implicated in a large number of food intolerances as well as triggering tinnitus for some. Unfortunately they can be tricky to avoid. Food containing high levels of salicylates include berries, oranges and tangerines, pineapples, peppers, tomatoes, green olives, almonds, peanuts, coconut oil, olive oil, processed meats, corn syrup, honey, jams, and dried fruits.

Unfortunately, alcoholic drinks such as red wine, grain-based spirits such as rum and beer, cider, sherry and brandy all contain high levels of salicylates so it's best to avoid them completely.

Additionally, salicylates are the main active ingredient in aspirin and often trigger tinnitus. If you remember, this is what started my tinnitus symptoms and they may affect yours too. It's best to avoid them and choose another kind of painkiller instead.

-Additives

Everyone knows what additives are and I'm pretty certain that you know that they are terrible for your health. But did you know that they can also trigger attacks of tinnitus? The worst offender is the artificial sweetener aspartame, followed by MSG (monosodium glutamate aka flavor enhancer). If you are eating a nutrient-dense real food diet as outlined earlier, you don't need to worry about these things as they are not naturally part of the human diet.

-Sugar

A prolonged exposure to high levels of sugar in the diet wreaks havoc on the human body and often results in long term damage. Unstable blood sugar levels are linked to an increase of tinnitus symptoms for many sufferers, so it's vital that we aim to keep our own blood sugar levels stable. Eat wholesome food and avoid processed, high fat, high sugar foods. Eat regularly and don't go for too long between meals. Eat healthy snacks and keep those attacks at bay.

Could you be suffering from a food intolerance or allergy?

Many tinnitus sufferers find that when they identify a food allergy or intolerance and avoid that food item completely, that their symptoms disappear. It's worth considering whether this is what is triggering your symptoms.

If you suspect a food intolerance or allergy, you have two options. You can book a food allergy test with a local practitioner, or follow an elimination diet where you avoid suspected food for a month and see if your symptoms improve. Then slowly reintroduce these foods whilst watching for reactions. Common sensitivities for the tinnitus sufferer include salicylates, wheat and dairy.

Supplements that might help

The body of a tinnitus sufferer is a body in crisis so it needs every last shred of support that you can give it. My favorite way to help support my health and 'cover all the bases' is to take a daily multivitamin and mineral.

It's also worth considering supplementing with Vitamin B complex. The B vitamins are all involved in ensuring the health of the nervous system as well as the efficient production of energy, especially Vitamin B_{12} and may make the difference between a frazzled nervous system and a calm one. It can be notoriously hard to consume adequate levels of B_{12} from the modern diet, especially if you are vegetarian, vegan or following a special diet, so give your body a helping hand and supplement.

STEP 4: Stress Reduction and Management

How stressed are you feeling right now on a scale of 1 to 10? Be honest with yourself.

Most of us operate under such chronic levels of stress that we no longer even consciously register it. Modern life can be such a rush and there are so many demands being made on you, so many obligations to be met and so much to do.

STOP!

This is no way to live your life. Stress will take over your life and impact upon your health if you let it.

It's also one of the most common causes of tinnitus symptoms. Sometimes chronic levels of stress can trigger it, sometimes stress simply makes it worse. Whatever the case, reducing our levels of stress will help calm our frazzled nervous system and help us to return to a state of calm, a healthy life and one that is, hopefully, tinnitus-free.

Even if reducing your levels of stress doesn't resolve your condition entirely, it will give you the tools to cope more effectively and begin to live your life again without its dark cloud looming over your head.

Here are our 7 easy steps to conquering your stress levels permanently.

1) Understand your condition.

Knowledge is power, so educate yourself about tinnitus. Investigate as far as your curiosity will take you and free yourself from needless worry. Then accept that you are suffering from tinnitus and then take steps to fight it. Don't wallow in self-pity, don't give up hope and don't sink into a deep, dark depression. A victim mentality like this will waste energy that could have been otherwise spent fighting this symptom, keep you locked into victim mentality and also prevent you from healing.

If you skipped the earlier part of the book dedicated to understanding tinnitus, go back and read it now. Instead of wasting energy on worrying, you can spend it on healing.

So be positive, challenge those negative emotions and move forward in your fight. We're all right here with you.

2) Simplify your life.

It's all too easy to live a cluttered life. And I'm not only talking about our physical possessions here. We believe it's virtuous to have a life packed-full of activities and obligations, without allowing ourselves the opportunity to simply 'be'. We even use *busy-ness* as a gauge of our value and importance. But this is utter nonsense and creates a life of chaos. Instead, aim to strip your life down to the essentials and enjoy the peace and clarity that comes with a calm life and calm surroundings.

So consider what things you love; what things really matter to you and your life. Don't think about what your family thinks, or your spouse, or your neighbors or kids. Think long and hard about what you value, what you want and what you dream of. Then foster as much of this in your life and strive for your dreams, whilst ditching the rest. This will free up so much more time to relax and so much more time to do what you really enjoy doing.

And finally, ask for help when you need it. There's no shame in asking, and people will be pleased to help and support you.

3) Sleep more.

Despite our best intentions, the majority of us often end up sleeping several hours less than we'd like to, and we often find ourselves sleep-deprived and using stimulants such as tea and coffee as crutches to help us survive the day. This is especially the case for us sufferers of tinnitus, as sleeping can often be close to impossible.
So make sleep a priority, and get as much of it as you can. You are not missing out on anything, only

promoting excellent health and reducing your tinnitus symptoms in the process. If you are having trouble sleeping due to your symptoms, read the next section on sound therapy and other therapies to discover some great tools you can use to relieve your problems.

4) Decompress.

It's essential that you claim some 'down time' for yourself to process the events of the day and to enjoy your life. You deserve it, you've earned it.

Foster some healthy habits that will allow yourself the space and opportunity to heal and get some relief from the demands and stresses of everyday life by indulging in whatever you like doing best. Maybe for you this is meditation or yoga, activities such as walking, time spent outside in the fresh air, exercise, starting a journal or taking relaxing baths.

Indulge in activities you love to do and your tinnitus symptoms should improve as well as your overall well-being.

5) Consider therapy.

Symptoms of stress are often a reflection of an inner emotional or psychological struggle that you are still dealing with.

Perhaps you've recently gone through a difficult time in your life such as a relationship break-up, a redundancy from work, losing a loved one or financial difficulties. Perhaps you had a difficult childhood or a traumatic experience somewhere along the way. Perhaps you were mercilessly bullied at school and have a hard time coming to terms with it and pulling your self-worth and confidence out the other side.

These things can impact upon your tinnitus, increase its severity or even trigger it in the first place. Our bodies often develop physical ailments in order to deal with inner pain. Don't ignore it any more. Look for ways to unpack your emotional issues, deal with grief and develop a positive outlook that will help you move forward in your life, and away from tinnitus. Do some research,and find a therapist near your home who can help you deal with the challenges that tinnitus can bring.

6) **Seek out support groups.**

When I was diagnosed, I thought I was alone in my suffering, and the powerlessness and loneliness was crippling. Then a concerned friend discovered a website that she thought might help. It was the site of a national support group that helps connect sufferers of tinnitus and share their stories, their experiences and lend a listening ear. This had such an incredible impact upon my life that I'd highly recommend it to anyone suffering from any kind of condition.

Having the support of someone who truly understands what you are going through made all of the difference to my quality of life; at last I realized that I was not alone and that people can and do get through it. There are hundreds of local groups (in the US and the world!), online support groups and forums that will help give you the support that you crave.

Look to the resources section for a list of groups that might help you.

7) **Eat healthily and cut out cigarettes and alcohol**

Diet and lifestyle habits greatly affect both our personal experience of stress and the impact that this stress has upon the body. Great nutrition has the power to support our bodies and minds through this difficult time. So do yourself a favor; eat healthily according to the guidelines above, quit alcohol and cut down on 'recreational' drugs and smoking to give your body and nervous system a chance to rest.

STEP 5: Sound therapy (and other therapies)

In this section we will concentrate on treatments that will help to instantly relieve your symptoms of tinnitus. Through their use you will sleep better, become less distracted, become more positive and motivated and finally enjoy a freedom from its torturous incessant sounds. They can be used individually together as part of a comprehensive treatment plan; do whatever works best for you.

Background noise

This is the simplest trick to use in reducing your tinnitus symptoms. Tinnitus often rears its ugly head and becomes more noticeable when your surroundings are quiet, such as at bedtime, in the bathroom, in the public library, when studying or when focusing on certain tasks.

Use background sounds such as music, the radio, the TV or even 'white' noise to conceal the tinnitus, reduce stress and distract you from your symptoms. If you suffer from a milder form, you may find this eliminates your symptoms all together.

Environmental sound generators

These devices emit continuous relaxing sounds of nature which will help mask your tinnitus symptoms so you can live a normal life, much in the same way as our background noise recommendation above. They are wonderful to use when falling asleep, and can really make the difference between a lousy night's sleep and a refreshing rejuvenating one. You can even get devices that are tailored for bedtime such as special 'pillow speakers' for night-time use. You can even get devices that fit onto your ear like a hearing aid, and many existing hearing aids have this technology inbuilt.

Tinnitus retraining therapy (TRT)

This is a therapy 'package' which combines sound therapy plus counseling for great overall relief. It gets you used to your tinnitus symptoms to such a degree that it no longer registers as part of your conscious but subconscious instead. In other words, you'll just 'get used to' those annoying sounds instead of being so affected by them.

CBT (cognitive behavioural therapy)

Cognitive behavioral therapy is not designed to eliminate your symptoms of tinnitus. What it will do is help you to deal with the impact that it has upon your life, and find ways of coping and feeling more positive about your prognosis.

Conclusion

Tinnitus is irritating, maddening and upsetting to live with. It can prevent you from living your life to its fullest, keep you in a constant state of sleep-deprivation and depression, but it needn't be a life sentence.

You **can** regain your personal power, loosen yourself from the iron grip of your symptoms and get back to normal again. And you will.

The key is education. Educate yourself as best you can about tinnitus using this great book. Understand its symptoms and its causes, and then vow to tackle your symptoms by using the tools we've gathered for you in this book: acceptance, optimum nutrition, stress-reduction, and sound & cognitive therapies.

Using the techniques in this book has enabled me to almost entirely relieve my tinnitus symptoms and quite literally save my life.

Just a few months ago I wouldn't have believed that this could be possible, but here I am, sharing my wisdom so that it can help others like you too. There was a lot of research, a lot of experimentation and a lot of trial and error along the way, and I feel so grateful and blessed that a true solution to our torturous symptoms really is out there.

Turn now to our resources section to find out contact details for some of the best tinnitus support groups and websites out there.

Thank you for allowing me to share my journey back to full health with me. I hope you enjoy your own healing process and live your life to its fullest. I know I intend to!

Resources

American Tinnitus Association http://www.ata.org/

Tinnitus UK http://www.tinnitus.org.uk/

Canadian Tinnitus Foundation
http://www.findthecurenow.org/

Australian Tinnitus Association
http://www.tinnitus.asn.au/

Tinnitus talk support forum http://www.tinnitustalk.com/

Tinnitus Support Message Board
http://www.tinnitusinfo.org/

Tinnitus Support Group: Facebook
https://www.facebook.com/TinnitusSupport